MAKE
WORLDS

CW00552975

To Christiane
from

Simon
Oli
Ross

Simon Taylor-Robinson,
Orli Rhodes Kendler, Ross Parker

The Antiviral Diet

europe books

© 2021 **Europe Books** | London
www.europebooks.co.uk – info@europebooks.co.uk

ISBN 979-12-201-0978-9
First edition: June 2021

Distribution for the United Kingdom: **Vine House Distribution ltd**

Printed for Italy by Rotomail Italia
Finito di stampare nel mese di giugno 2021
presso Rotomail Italia S.p.A. - Vignate (MI)

The Antiviral Diet

Acknowledgements

We are grateful to Graham Martin from Graham Martin Photography, London, United Kingdom (www. grahammartinphotography.co.uk) for all the photographic figures and to Eran Kendler for all the illustrative diagrams in the book.

PART 1

Health and Nutrients

WHAT THE BODY NEEDS

It is often said that "you are what you eat", but although this has been cast aside by millions of people without a second thought, never a truer maxim was coined. All living beings have to detoxify, replenish, grow and repair – and where does that life force come from?

It comes from what we eat.

For the most part, **food** is made of three types: **carbohydrates** (standard energy givers), **proteins** (the main building blocks of the body) and **fats** (needed for the membranes of our **body cells** with certain fats important for the immune system and also brain function).

Figure 1 illustrates types of dietary carbohydrate (such as bread, rice, pasta and potatoes), protein (such as meat, fish, tofu and nuts) and fats (such as butter, margarine and olive oil). Our diet is composed of a mixture of all of them and many foods or food dishes are complex, containing protein, fat, and carbohydrate together.

Probably the best known of the carbohydrates is **sugar**. There are a number of different sugars – **fructose** is present naturally in fruits with some fruits having much more in the way of sugar content than others. Generally, it is true that tropical fruits have a higher fructose content than fruits grown in temperate or colder climates, which is important when one considers diabetes (a condition where the body's sugar control is impaired). The amount of sugar present in fruit, for example, is indicated in the **"glycemic index"**. A high glycemic index indicates a food with a lot of sugar, whereas a lower glycemic index indicates a food with less sugar. This is particularly important to note for people with **diabetes**, where blood sugar control is a problem.

The sugar that we are most familiar with is **sucrose**, which is what we put in our tea or coffee. It comes from sugar cane or sugar beet and is notorious for causing dental cavities, although originally it was so highly prized that Queen Elizabeth I of England in the 16th Century was said to have actually brushed her teeth in it! However, nowadays, we know that sugary foods add to the problem of the obesity epidemic of modern man and also we now know that it has adverse effects on our immune system.

However, too much in the way of alternatives, such as artificial sweeteners, is not great either for a healthy and balanced body. **So, when can we have sugar?** Generally, it is better to have sugar in a meal and avoid it as a snack. Later in the book, we have a section on healthy desserts!

Along the theme of being made up of what we eat (for better or worse), **Figure 2** shows a picture of a cell – these are the building blocks of the body. Each cell is involved in energy metabolism and is composed of phospholipid (a type of complex fat), the sources of which, we get mainly from our diet. Therefore, to have a healthy body, we need a varied and healthy diet.

Figure 1 - Figure 1 Type of Dietary Carbohydrate, Protein and Fats

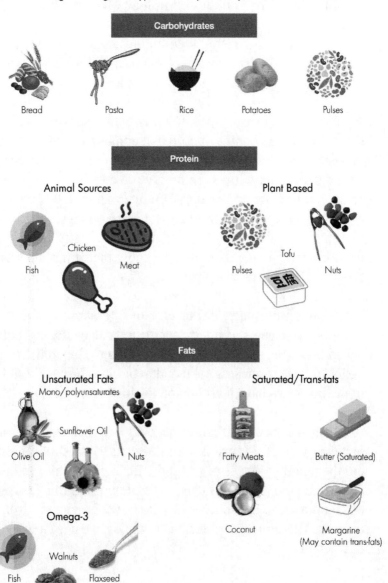

Figure 2 - The Cell

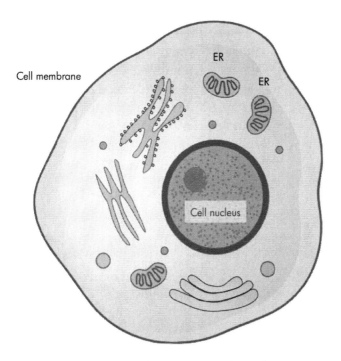

The cell contains both internal and external membranes that are made up of phospholipids which are largely composed of fats. Some of these internal structures are involved in energy metabolism - endoplasmic reticulum (ER)

In addition to the carbohydrates, proteins, and fats in the diet, we also need **vitamins**, which are essential for normal bodily performance and play a vital role in immune function. **Table 1** shows the different vitamins and what they are needed for – and also what foods are good sources of each vitamin.

The need for **vitamin C** became known in the early days of the British Empire, when British sailors on long voyages at sea became ill with a disease called scurvy (caused by vitamin C deficiency). Their diet was usually based on sea biscuits, but it was noticed that a squeeze of lime into the rum rations prevented the illness. The practice became widespread through the Navy and is the reason why British servicemen were known as "limeys". Since then, it has been well accepted that all citrus fruits have enough vitamin C in them to prevent scurvy – a disease which should never be seen these days if people have a healthy diet. It is important to note that a diet that has enough vitamin C is important for a healthy immune system and for good wound healing, regeneration, and repair of the body.

Folic acid is another very important vitamin and the key to a good immune system; pregnant women, in particular, are advised to consume a recommended intake of folic acid because it is critical for the development of the unborn baby and for the development of a healthy nervous system and brain.

Vitamin D is an interesting vitamin because a lot of it is made in the skin in the presence of sunlight, but the rest is obtained from the diet. Many people in countries with long winter nights, such as in northern Europe, are vitamin D deficient, particularly in the winter, owing to a lack of sunlight. It is important to be aware of this because vitamin D is extremely important for a healthy immune system and to fight viral illnesses. In the context of the COVID-19 pandemic, vitamin D supplementation is often given to help fight the virus in those who are deficient, but it is important to remember that some foods are a good source of it – such as eggs, liver, and oily fish.

If one tips **fibre** into the mix for normal **gut action**, we have the components of human diets, which have generally been unaltered over the centuries until the modern transport system radically changed the availability of food, going from a society based on seasonal foods to a society where anything is accessible all the time.

Figure 3 - Digestive System

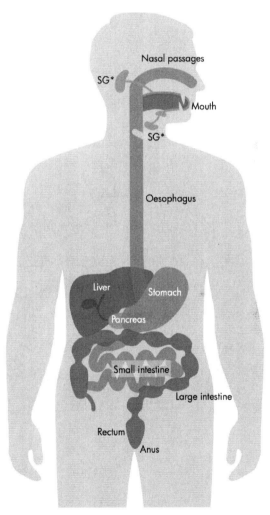

*SG = salivary gland

The human body has a complex **digestive system (Figure 3)** which is designed to break down food into soluble components that can be absorbed easily into the body across the surface of the gut and on into the bloodstream, so that we can use the components for body repair, growth, and replenishment.

Figure 4 - Functions of the Liver

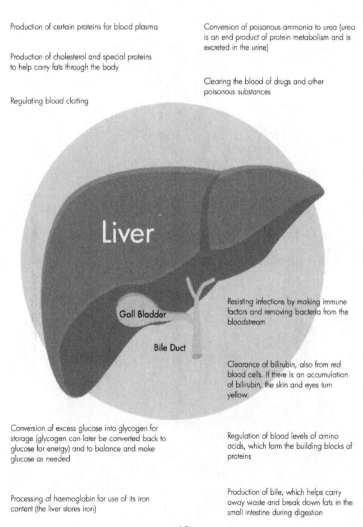

Production of certain proteins for blood plasma

Production of cholesterol and special proteins to help carry fats through the body

Regulating blood clotting

Conversion of poisonous ammonia to urea (urea is an end product of protein metabolism and is excreted in the urine)

Clearing the blood of drugs and other poisonous substances

Resisting infections by making immune factors and removing bacteria from the bloodstream

Clearance of bilirubin, also from red blood cells. If there is an accumulation of bilirubin, the skin and eyes turn yellow.

Conversion of excess glucose into glycogen for storage (glycogen can later be converted back to glucose for energy) and to balance and make glucose as needed

Regulation of blood levels of amino acids, which form the building blocks of proteins

Processing of haemoglobin for use of its iron content (the liver stores iron)

Production of bile, which helps carry away waste and break down fats in the small intestine during digestion

16

Some of the nutrients circulate to repair and renew muscles, bones, and internal body organs, while others are either stored in the liver or used as an energy source by the liver to clear away toxins that have built up in our body. These impurities may be from the natural decomposition of our cells in the course of everyday bodily breakdown and renewal, or from what we eat or take into our bodies in the form of medicines or dietary impurities. The liver plays a vital role in keeping a balance in the body: making proteins from dietary building blocks for cell regeneration, and ensuring that blood and body are cleared of unwanted and harmful compounds. **Figure 4** shows the various function of the liver in an everyday healthy life.

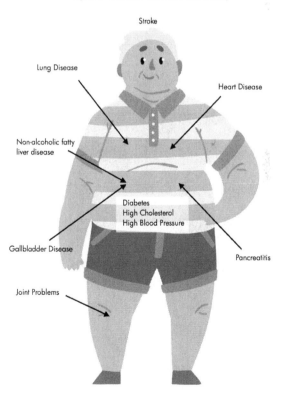

Figure 5 - Diseases Associated with Obesity

Stroke

Lung Disease

Heart Disease

Non-alcoholic fatty liver disease

Diabetes
High Cholesterol
High Blood Pressure

Gallbladder Disease

Pancreatitis

Joint Problems

Eating too much and doing little exercise leads to being overweight and obesity. Excessive dietary carbohydrates, in particular, if not consumed through exercise or activities, get stored in the body as fat, either under the surface of the skin or wrapped around the organs (so-called "visceral fat") – even if we do not eat much fat itself in our diet. **Fat** is the easiest source of energy to burn in case of fasting or famine, but too much fat is associated with disease in every part of the body, including the immune system.

Figure 5 shows all the diseases associated with obesity. It can be seen that obesity can cause diseases in almost every organ in the body, in addition to having an effect on the immune system and increasing the susceptibility to developing certain cancers too.

Figure 6 - What is a Virus

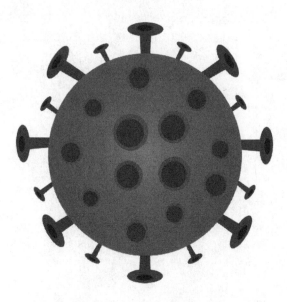

Viruses contain either a piece of DNA or RNA genetic material with an envelope made of protein. They are not alive, but are capable of reproducing themselves by getting into a cell, and hijacking normal cell function to produce further copies of themselves.

The immune system is composed of different types of white cells that circulate in the blood with a monitoring role, checking that the body is safe from potential invaders such as viruses.

Figure 6 shows a schematic of what a virus is. Essentially, viruses are fragments of genetic material encased in an envelope made chiefly of protein. Strangely, they are not living organisms (which are made up of cells), but they do have the ability to reproduce themselves, using much of the machinery present in living cells (Figure 2), which they hijack to perform functions that the virus needs. Once they have done this in one individual, viruses may infect another person and use the new, healthy cells to reproduce again.

Our immune system is designed to prevent viruses from gaining entry, but it may not always be effective. We may need additional protection from viral vaccines, and/or from natural antiviral agents that are present in our diet and which stimulate the immune system to act more effectively.

Figure 7 - Conditions predisposing to Viral Illness

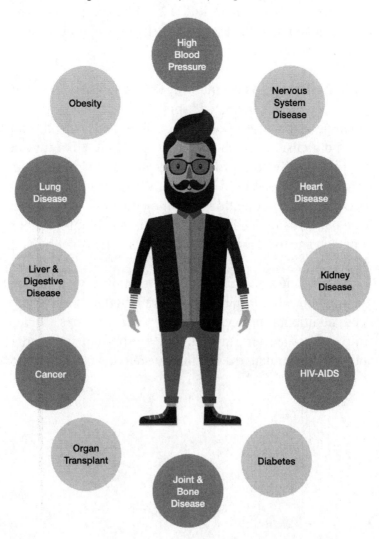

When the body gets attacked by an outside agent like a virus, a healthy immune system comes into play to try to neutralise the invader and minimise any damage done. This is done very successfully in most cases, but some people with certain conditions may fight viruses and other invaders less efficiently. Such conditions include obesity and diabetes. **Figure 7** shows certain conditions predisposing to viral illnesses.

Figure 8 - Components of a Healthy Diet

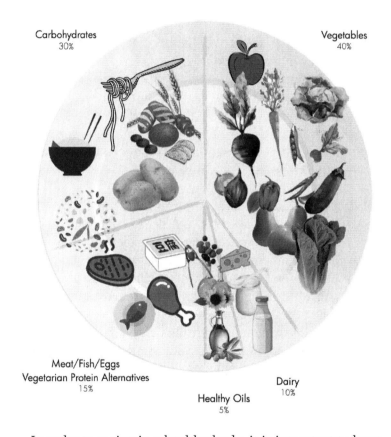

Carbohydrates
30%

Vegetables
40%

Meat/Fish/Eggs
Vegetarian Protein Alternatives
15%

Dairy
10%

Healthy Oils
5%

In order to maintain a healthy body, it is important to have a **healthy diet**, which is not overloaded with carbohydrates, has a good proportion of protein from meat, fish and/or vegetables for body renewal, while remembering that some fats are good for us, including the so-called "essential fatty acids".

There is no magic to eating well – we were designed to be hunter-gatherers and our ancestors lived on seasonal foods. They were not subject to obesity or the excesses of modern life, but ate small amounts of food often and combined this with regular physical exercise. **Figure 8** shows the components of a healthy diet.

In addition to a healthy balanced diet, we also have to consider the **environment** in which we live. We should live in harmony with our work, home, and leisure components of our life, but this can be very difficult to achieve. Unfortunately, **stress** has an effect on everything we do and on the equilibrium and balance in our body. If there is too much stress, it can have an effect on our immune system and on how we fight illnesses, including viruses.

What is stress? Well, it is a state of heightened alert which we used as primitive cavemen in order to hunt animals or to run away when there was danger. The body uses certain hormones, such as adrenaline and cortisol, which we produce to quicken the pace of the heart, to send blood to the muscles in order to run after an animal or run away from danger. However, in modern life, our brains can perceive work environments as emotionally dangerous with the same "fight" or "flight" hormones released, despite the fact that we are not running anywhere and are not in any immediate danger.

An excessive amount of stress hormones can end up in the development of a series of diseases including heart disease and high blood pressure, which can lead to strokes and other diseases typical of the modern-day stressed person. However, adopting a healthy diet and a regular exercise routine allows that stress to be mitigated, although it has to be said that we all function on a certain degree of stress to get out of bed every day (actually our stress hormones are naturally at their highest in the early morning when we do get up).

There is clearly an optimal level of stress to allow the body to function normally and for a balanced life and a good, reactive immune system. However, striking that balance is something that needs individual tuning, but in this book, we hope to bring some tips on healthy diet and exercise in the era of a viral pandemic.

Figure 9- High Fructose and Lactose Containing Products

The following are examples of foods high in Fructose or Lactose

Fructose			
Apples		Onion	
Pears		Leek	
Fruit Juice		Garlic	
Honey		Asparagus	
Lactose			
Cheese		Milk	
Cream		Ice Cream	

Some people are less able to absorb certain components of the diet than others. Sometimes these **dietary intolerances** (or **malabsorption**) run in families. Two of the commonest problems are a failure to absorb lactose, the sugar present in dairy products, and a failure to absorb fructose, the sugar present in fruits (**Figure 9** – high fructose and lactose-containing products). If someone has such intolerances, these sugars do not get absorbed easily and end up causing abdominal discomfort, bloating, tummy rumbling, wind, and diarrhoea.

Table 1 - Vitamin Function

Viatamin	Function	Sources
Thiamin (B1)	Energy metabolism, nerve function	Meat, wholegrain, vegetables, nuts, seeds
Riboflavin (B2)	Energy metabolism, vision, healthy skin	Dairy products, leafy greens, wholegrain
Niacin (B3)	Energy metabolism, digestive, skin, nerve health	Meat, poultry, wholegrain, mushrooms, vegetables - asparagus, leafy greens, peanuts
Pantothenic Acid	Energy metabolism	Widespread in foods
Biotin	Energy metabolism	Widespread in foods and produced by gut bacteria
Pyridoxine (B6)	Protein metabolism, red blood cell manufacture	Meat, fish, vegetables, fruit
Folic Acid	Cell health including red blood cells	Leafy greens, legumes, seeds, liver, wholegrain
Cobalamin (B12)	Cell health and nerve function	Meat, fish, seafood, eggs, dairy products
Ascorbic Acid (C)	Antioxidant, protein metabolism, immune health, iron absorption	Fruit and vegetables
Vitamin A (Precursor - Beta Carotene)	Healthy vision, skin, bones, teeth, immune system	Dairy products, eggs, liver. Betacarotene - leafy dark greens, apricots, melons, carrots, squash, sweet potatoes, pumpkins
Vitamin D	Calcium absorption, bone health, immune health	Eggs, liver, oily fish (Sunlight - made in skin)
Vitamin E	Antioxidant, cell health	Polyunsaturated oils: soya, corn, cottonseed, safflower; leafy green, wheatgerm, wholegrain, liver, eggs nuts, seeds
Vitamin K	Blood clotting	Leafy greens (kale, spinach), broccoli, Brussels sprouts, asparagus (also made by gut bacteria)

Vitamins A, D, E and K are fat soluble, the rest being water soluble

Another common food intolerance is to **gluten**, which is a protein component of wheat, barley, and to a lesser extent, oats. **Gluten sensitivity** is not as common as many people think. It causes a malabsorption condition called **coeliac disease**, which is quite uncommon. However, if you think you have problems with wheat-based products, your doctor can arrange a simple blood test to check.

Therefore, there is always some difference in what is good for each individual, but in a world that is coming to terms with a global viral pandemic, we give some simple ideas on eating well to help our immune system, while maintaining exercise in simple ways that allow us to be fit, even if we have to stay indoors. Our aim is to enable you, the reader, through knowledge and some simple examples, to springboard yourself to a healthier lifestyle.

We enjoy our food for both its taste and the social aspect of preparing and eating it, but the way we make food and combine the different elements of the meal can have a profound effect on our health. We need to try and take control of what we put on our plate, so we can keep on enjoying food while maximising the health benefits of our food intake – you will find that this actually doesn't take much effort, but just a bit of knowledge and attention.

One size doesn't fit all
We are constantly asked very valid questions, such as:
– Should I eat breakfast?
– Should I have a big meal at lunch or dinner?
– What exercise should I do?

We wish we could give a simple answer that will fit everyone who is reading this, but the unfortunate truth is that one size doesn't fit all – we need to find the answers which suit our body, tastes, and lifestyle. Don't worry – the good news is that this is easily achievable.

A BALANCED DIET

The body needs a balanced dietary intake in order to function properly and to have a healthy immune system. This means having a balanced intake of carbohydrates, proteins, and fats. It should be noted that we need some of everything in our diet and that, although often thought of as bad, there really are good fats which are vital for a healthy functioning body, including the joints, the brain, and the immune system.

Most drugs in the Western medical compendium are derived from plant extracts, either directly or indirectly, so it stands to reason that a diet rich in certain foods can help us maintain health and help in our fight against certain viruses, like COVID-19.

In this chapter, we look at a healthy, balanced diet with seasonal foods and take a look at some foods that act as natural antiviral agents.

Natural antivirals: Vitamin C, folic acid, vitamin D and zinc

These vitamins and minerals have all been recommended as useful immune-boosting agents in the diet. **Vitamin C** is a large component of citrus fruits, as most people know, but also present in vegetables, including potatoes. **Folic acid** takes its name from the Latin term for leaf, and is present in leafy green vegetables, such as kale, spinach and cabbage. **Zinc** is present in whole grains, beans, chickpeas, nuts, and red meat, while many breakfast cereals have zinc added. Most people in temperate climates do not receive enough **vitamin D** from sunshine and it is difficult to supplement the deficit from diet only, so many people need to take supplements on a daily basis to maintain proper levels of vitamin D (NHS guidelines of 10 micrograms per day). Other natural antivirals include **quercetin**, which is a "flavonoid", commonly found in berries, such as blueberries, blackberries and raspberries.

Natural anti-inflammatory agents

These include purple fruit and vegetables, all of which are high in **lycopene**. Examples include blueberries, blackberries, blackcurrants, black grapes, beetroot and red cabbage. As a general guideline, it is sensible to use a handful of each, as long as you get variety.

The following herbs and plants have either antiviral effects or immune-stimulating properties:

Herbs:

Oregano – contains the antiviral carvacrol

Sage – contains safficinolide, a natural antiviral

Basil and **Tulsi** – contains apigenin and ursolic acid, immune boosters

Fennel – contains trans-anethole, a natural antiviral

Garlic – antiviral activity in addition to being good for blood pressure and an immune cell booster

28

Lemon Balm – potential effect against influenza

Peppermint – contains menthol and rosmarinic acid which have antiviral activity and anti-inflammatory activity

Rosemary – contains oleanolic acid which has some antiviral activity according to laboratory studies

Echinacea – antiviral and immune-boosting effects

Elderberry – antiviral and immune-stimulating properties

Licorice – contains glycyrrhizin, liquiritigenin, and glabridin that have antiviral properties, recognised from Chinese medicine – said to have been effective in SARS.

Ginger – contains gingerols and zingerone which inhibit viral replication and prevent viruses from entering host cells, in laboratory studies.

Ginseng – contains ginsenosides which have antiviral activity according to laboratory studies.

Dandelion – antiviral activity according to laboratory studies too.

It should be remembered that most of the drugs and medical treatments that we have today have either a direct or indirect origin in herbs and plants which were used by traditional medicine in days gone by. Such examples include aspirin, which was first obtained from a tree bark. Herbs remain important for their medicinal qualities, in addition to being flavourful for our food.

It is true that in modern times, we are losing the knowledge of what is growing around us and how to use it. Rather than relying on dried herbs, we would encourage everyone to have some pots of herbs at home, so as to experience their smells and fresh flavour. We still need to consider taking some natural remedies, so why not include them in food through the use of herbs? A lot of sensible dietary remedies have been lost in modern day society, but it is not too late to ask your elders to write down family traditions!

Care must be taken not to stray from the basics of a **balanced diet**. Beetroot, for example, has been touted in the media as a cure-all for anything and everything, but it has a very high sugar load, in the form of fructose, which can be a problem in those who do not absorb that sugar easily.

Eating Habits

It is important not to eat for the sake of it, just because it is mealtime. Eating if you feel hungry is a good maxim. The important thing for the body is **not to overeat** just because food is there. Leaving some food on the plate for another time is not a sin, despite the thoughts of post-war austerity that often linger.

However, many people take a rushed attitude to their meals. It is good for the body and for the immune system for us all to sit down **at a table**, to take time to enjoy the sight, smell, and taste of food and let the body digest a meal with time. This also allows the body to receive and process the food we have eaten in the most effective way. **Eating too fast** often leads to over-eating and conversely, to a rise

30

in blood sugars that may be harmful to some. The advice is to **take time** to eat small amounts sensibly and regularly at a table, rather than in front of a computer, tablet, phone, or television.

Taking time to **chew food** properly is important – the very process reports back to the brain that we are eating. As the gut and the brain communicate with each other in something called "the gut-brain axis", signals are sent to the brain to say that we are eating - it actually helps a feeling of fulness or well-being (so-called "satiety") if we chew well. Many people do not know that there are digestive enzymes in our saliva (so-called "salivary amylases"), which are there to aid digestion, but they are hardly given time to work if we eat our food too quickly. Spending time to eat and chewing deliberately is what we were designed to do and it helps our general stress balance if we remember that.

If we are stressed, certain stress hormones, such as cortisol, increase in the blood and this has a direct effect on the immune system, often in a bad way. So relaxing, allowing the brain to take in the sight, smell and taste of food allows us to gain the maximum from what we eat.

Mealtimes are important. As we said before, the body is at its most alert and needy in the early morning (when there are high levels of the hormone, cortisol, which is needed to get us up and active for the day). It is at this point that having a good breakfast is important, as the body is primed and ready to repair and regenerate using the food eaten. It used to be said, "Eat breakfast like a king", but in today's society, there are some who have lost sight of this in the hurry to get on with their daily lives.

It is also true that in days gone by lunch used to be a

bigger affair than it is today for the busy working person, and that dinner was not the main meal of the day. Actually, eating late at night is bad for us in many ways, including the fact that our cortisol levels are at their lowest and the body is least primed to receive food and use it for regeneration and regrowth. Going to bed on a full stomach is not the best policy for our metabolism and for a healthy balance. If it can be managed, eating earlier is helpful, rather than presenting a lot of food to our system just before we go to bed (when the body needs to rest, rather than work to digest food efficiently and effectively).

Portion size and appearance of the plate

So many times we have been asked:
"How much should I have?"
"What is a portion size, and how many times a week?"
"What can I have it with and how to make it?"

Portions depend on body size, but a good guide is that a plate should contain a fist-sized portion of carbohydrates such as rice or potatoes, a fist-sized portion of meat or fish, and two fist-sized portions of vegetables. A healthy diet should have a rainbow of colors with green, purple, orange, yellow, and red fruit and vegetables. If we want to lose weight, as a general rule, then the portion of vegetables should be bigger and the carbohydrate portion smaller.

The psychology of food

Supermarkets are encouraging us to buy more food in jumbo packs, "buy-one-get-one-free" offers, special promotions, price reductions, and product placement at supermarket tills. We are all under pressure, overt or otherwise, to buy more than we need and thus to eat it. However, restraint is needed as a substantial proportion of what we buy spoils and is never eaten, either because of incorrect storage, limited shelf lives, or simply because we buy too much.

A useful way to practice restraint is to look at the ingredients on the back of a food packet and to learn to look at the calorie content, the saturated fat content, and the numbers of preservatives. This allows us to make informed choices and sometimes to put what we have selected back on the supermarket shelf!

Another way to practice restraint is to have a **shopping list** and keep to it, rather than being tempted to buy in an impulsive way whatever looks appealing in the special offer aisle of the supermarket. It goes without saying that we shouldn't go shopping in the supermarket when we are hungry, as the temptation is there to come back with a lot of unnecessary things, including unhealthy snacks!

A healthy approach

The use of local markets, looking at **seasonal foods** is a healthy approach because they are generally locally grown, and higher in nutrients such as vitamin C because these foods (root vegetables in the winter, salads in the summer, for example) usually have less storage time from farm to the plate. A benefit is that seasonal foods are fresher and retain the nutrients for longer.

Historically, it was the rich who ate unhealthy diets, overloaded with carbohydrates and fat. One just has to think of the Georgian and Victorian periods with pictures of gouty men and excessively rich foods. It is healthy perhaps to look back on the peasant diet of the time, which was full of freshly grown vegetables, fruits, and **whole grains**. What was good for us in the past still holds today!

Processed foods may be cheaper, but they are not necessarily healthier. Equally well, the obsession with **fruit juices** leads to very high sugar loads, which contributes to being overweight, because it takes a considerable number of oranges to make one glass of juice. From a digestive point of view, it is better to chew a single orange and benefit from the **fibre** contained in it, which then contributes to a regular bowel movement without the excessive sugar load.

Eating on a budget

It is not difficult to eat healthily on a budget because canned and frozen food still contains good nutrients. Canned fish is high in essential oils, while frozen berries, for example, add an easy topping to porridge at breakfast time and remain high in vitamin C and quercetin. It is important also to remember that many delicious recipes can be made from leftovers to stretch a budget – such as soups, pies, stir-fries, and curries. We give a few healthy options later on in the book.

Foods to consider for a healthy immune-boosting and antiviral diet:

- Avocado
- Walnuts
- Almonds
- Pine nuts
- Oregano
- Camomile

- Carrots
- Olive oil
- Whole grains
- Sunflower seeds
- Mustard
- Coriander
- Jasmine
- Cumin
- Saffron
- Lemon
- Fresh mint
- Thyme
- Sage
- Tomatoes
- Lentils
- Parsley
- Chilli
- Cinnamon
- Rosemary
- Pomegranate
- Fennel
- Sesame
- Oats
- Oily fish
- Lean meat

A short, but digestible (pun intended) explanation of the science of food

All foods are a combination of 'Macro' and 'Micro' nutrients

Don't hide under the table yet – it's much simpler than you think…

Macronutrients are 'the big' building blocks of our food:

– **Protein** such as eggs, pulses, nuts, meat
– **Carbohydrates** ("carbs") such as bread, cereal, rice, pasta, pastry, potatoes
– **Fats** such as oils, cheese, nuts
You may think that each food item will belong just to one of the above three, but in reality, the majority of foods are actually a combination of the three.

Oats, for example, are mostly associated with carbohydrates, but actually they are a very good source of protein (almost 17%) and fat (almost 7%). Avocados, on the other hand, might be known as a good source of protein, but they have 9% of carbohydrate in their make-up.

There are some foods that are predominantly one of the three elements. Oil is pure fat, while granulated sugar is pure carbohydrate, but you will find that most other dietary components are a combination of these three elements.

Why is this so important to know? This is because there is a lot of misinformation about what we eat, and of what we should be eating more or less.

Let's look at protein for example
Our body is a very clever machine. You can get enough protein from either animal products or a combination of pulses, vegetables, and meat alternatives.

We are designed to make protein from smaller components called amino acids: these combine together to supply us with the protein we need, so a varied diet will provide enough building blocks to avoid any deficiencies, and hence allow our body to make the necessary protein it needs for growth and maintenance.

Let's talk about fat…

This subject again has a lot of misinformation surrounding it, yet it is quite simple to understand.

There are three types of fat:

– **Saturated fats** such as butter and fat from meats. These tend to be **solid** at room temperature. For a variety of health reasons, saturated fats should only be consumed in moderation.

– **Mono-** and **Poly-unsaturated** fats such as olive oil and sunflower oil are liquid at room temperature, and while slightly different, they both are essential for our diets and considered better for our health than saturated fats.

Every fat has a slightly different melting point, so some fats, although they are very healthy uncooked, may not be suitable for frying food at a high temperature.

Let's move on to 'Micro' nutrients

This is an 'umbrella' term to describe the combination of vitamins and minerals that our body desperately needs for growth, brain development, and immunity amongst others. While our body needs a smaller amount of these to function (hence the term 'micro'), it cannot produce these by itself. A healthy and balanced diet can easily provide our body with most of the required micronutrients we need.

We haven't changed – the world has

Our bodies have not changed over the past hundreds and thousands of years. What has changed are both our lifestyle and the way food is presented to us. We don't need to hunt anymore, we mostly live a sedentary lifestyle and food is readily available in packaged form where we may have absolutely no clue of what is contained inside the box. And if that's not stressful enough, our jobs are ever more complicated, leaving little time for well thought out diet and exercise – with the temptation to go for the easy and often unhealthy option.

Our relationship with food has changed from food being a necessity to recreational and even social activity. While we can continue to enjoy food, we also need to understand that food can have both positive and negative impacts on our health. With a few simple rules and a positive attitude, we can continue to enjoy our meals and stay healthy for much longer.

10 Simple Rules:

– The Plate Model (see Figure 8, page 21); a variety of constituents represented on the plate
– Not just what we eat, but how we eat
– Eating times
– Mix and match food constituents, but remembering the basics
– Shopping right
– Portion size
– Variety
– Gut flora
– Exercise
– A good night sleep

So it is important to remember a plate with colorful fruit and vegetables, taking time to eat at a table at regular times, a balance between protein, carbohydrate and some fat, shopping for seasonal ingredients, not over-eating, having foods that help the good bacteria in our gut (gut flora), together with some exercise and a good night's sleep. Does it sound easy? Well, with a bit of training, it is!

The thing about a healthy diet is to remember **the basics** and realize that with a few simple ingredients, an interesting, varied and healthy diet can be built up.

Perhaps, last but least, we need to mention that our gut is home to billions and billions of bacteria which live in harmony with us. These gut bacteria are termed "**the microbiome**". They aid the digestion of the food we eat and actually help us absorb nutrients from the gut – they are such an important part of who and what we are, as everybody's normal population of gut bacteria is different.

The gut bacteria are vital for maintaining a healthy immune system, but for example, if we are ill or when we take antibiotics unnecessarily, the populations of gut bacteria can be altered or diminished. The use of probiotic foods, such as those that can be found in the yoghurt counter of the supermarket, can help restore a normal and healthy gut bacteria population again – as our resident population soon bounces back when we are healthy.

Some foods promote a healthy gut microbiome, such as green vegetables, fish, and dietary fibre. Having a balanced diet with diversity helps maintain a healthy microbiome. As we get older we lose some of the diversity of the microbiome and this makes us more open to disease processes. It is therefore important to be aware of a healthy, diverse diet, as we discuss in the next chapter.

PART 2

Food and Recipes

How many times did you buy a cookbook and only use it once or twice? Don't despair… you are not alone.

It is said that we only ever use ten recipes in our lifetime. Once we become more confident, we learn to improvise, and become more adventurous with the ingredients we use in these recipes.

This is exactly what our goal is. We want to give you some easy and fun ideas. Choose the ones you like, and then feel free to change, experiment, and push yourself outside your comfort zone.

We want you to experiment with different herbs and spices. Flavours you remember from your childhood or even borrowed from your favourite restaurants or friends are all good. Grow herbs on your window ledge, in a pot, or in your garden. Explore your local markets to find seasonal food and new foods you have never seen before.

Recipe books can be used as guidelines. Look at what inspires you and what would you like to try. Don't worry about swapping ingredients, if you don't try you will never know.

There is, however, something very important that we would like you to consider. We urge you to find out where your food is coming from, how it is grown, and when is it in season.

Seasonal food is fresh and provides you with the nutrients that are needed for your health. Eating a variety of foods in season should provide you with all the nutrients that you need. For example, during the winter, including root vegetables in your diet can be a good source of vitamin C. Having a variety of foods in your diet will help you reach the recommended daily amounts that you need for optimal health. Furthermore, eating seasonal and local will also help you to reduce carbon footprint and support local farmers.

Food for thought (pun intended)

– Once you have mastered cooking fish, chicken, or meat and meat alternatives such as tofu, feel free to mix and match.

– You can keep it simple, bake or grill, add your preferred sauce or simply add some pesto.

– Always remember one simple rule: if you have plenty of color on your plate you are likely to reach your daily intake of nutrients.

– Exchange some recipes with friends: part of the joy of eating is thinking about how to make your food, it is simply the spice of life.

Know your food

We are very fortunate to live in a global village accessible by technology and widely available to us. As a result, we have much more access to a huge variety of food and ingredients that might have been ignored by previous generations or have been forgotten.

In the recipes outlined later on, you might find some ingredients that are not familiar to you, but don't let this hold you back. We hope you will find some new and exciting foods, that will be your "go-to" ingredients and "must-have" foods.

Nuts and **seeds** are a healthy option for both your diet and as a snack between meals should you feel hungry. They are a good source of fibre and polyunsaturated oils.

Each day:

– Try and have at least ten almonds: they are a good source of calcium and zinc.
– Two Brazil nuts, which are a good source of selenium.
– Walnuts are a good source of magnesium, and vitamin B-6.

Seeds are a great topping to add to sweet or savoury dishes, such as yoghurt, salads, soups, and casserole. You can also mix into breadcrumbs to add an extra dimension to a crusty topping.

If you enjoy experimenting or making your own bread or pasta, why not try some of the **ancient grains** that can be found in supermarkets? **Kamut** flour is a wonderful alternative when making bread: it is high in fibre, but has a nuttier creamier flavour.

Amaranth and **quinoa** are both a wonderful addition to our diet. They are high in protein and minerals, can be served hot or cold and are a great alternative to rice, or couscous. They are also gluten-free (see gluten sensitivity in the health section earlier).

Pulses – such as **chickpeas, lentils** and a variety of **beans** – are the dry, edible seeds of the legume family.

Try to have more pulses in your diet. These are easy to include in many dishes. If you don't have time to cook them yourself, try to have a variety of canned or ready-cooked pulses, which are readily available in many shops and supermarkets. You can add pulses to salads, soups, or as a standalone snack.

Pulses are good source of energy and protein. They also have some wonderful properties ("phyto chemicals"), which can help reduce cholesterol for example.

Putting it all together

While we have included some amazing recipes that are tried and tested in the next section, there are some very simple things you can introduce to your daily routine and meal preparations, that will enhance your health and enrich your taste buds. You don't have to follow everything to the letter, just take some ideas and implement them as you go along, and feel free to improvise and create your own recipes based on the knowledge you have acquired. Food is essential for your health but it's also lots of fun.

– Breakfast

A few ideas to start our day on a positive note; foods that can provide us with energy to get us through the morning...

Making Porridge:
Add oats and milk to the desired consistency.
You can also add:
– Chia seeds
– Nuts
– Pumpkin or flax seeds
– Berries such as blueberries, you can also use frozen berries
– Cinnamon
If you are in a rush you can **prepare it the night before** and keep it in the fridge.
This can also be taken to work or warmed up as a hot porridge.

Alternatives to sugar are:
– Rice syrup or rice malt syrup (fructose free)
– Maple syrup (low in fructose)
– Try and avoid granulated sugar where possible: you can reduce your dependence on it slowly.

Bread:
Try to have whole-meal wholegrain bread, seeded, or other high fibre options...

Types of spreads:
– Avocado
– Smoked Salmon
– Peanut, almond, cashew, or any other nut butter
– Sliced banana

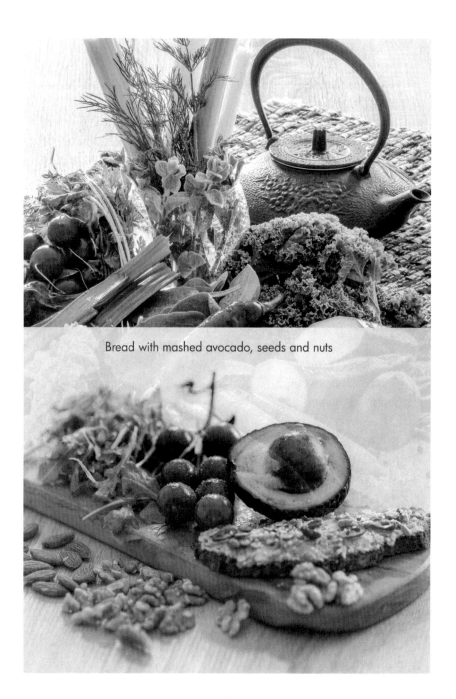

Bread with mashed avocado, seeds and nuts

Eggs

Eggs are versatile and can be made into a variety of dishes in any shape or form.

Enjoy a simple boiled egg, or have them scrambled, fried, or as an omelette.

A shakshuka makes a complete dish as it will have plenty of vegetables.

Green shakshuka: See recipe called "Green eggs, no ham"

Red shakshuka: Use the recipe for the green eggs, but replace green vegetables with red vegetables, such as tomatoes, and peppers.

Spanish omelette: this is a great way to combine eggs and potatoes: simply add cooked potatoes into fluffy beaten eggs, fry together with your favourite vegetables, such as courgettes (zucchini), peppers, or tomatoes.

Yoghurt

Natural, live – add fruit or cereal – also see our recipe for homemade granola.

– Lunch or Dinner

Try to have **fish** 3 times a week

It is best to have oily fish two of these times, as the oils needed for brain and immune function are found in high concentration in these types of fish.

Examples of oily fish: Salmon, trout, mackerel, fresh tuna, swordfish, herring, sardines, pilchards.

Meat and fish preparation

Always cut off visible fat from the meat before cooking. If you leave the fat on, it will melt and dissolve into your cooking. The same applies to removing the skin off the chicken prior to cooking as fat is stored under the skin. The exceptions are the fish that provide you with essential fatty acids.

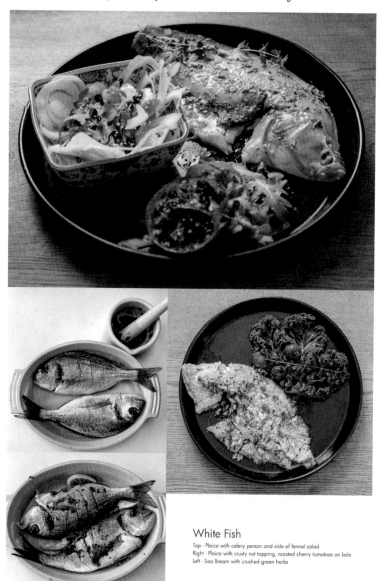

White Fish
Top - Plaice with celery person and side of fennel salad
Right - Plaice with crusty nut topping, roasted cherry tomatoes on kale
Left - Sea Bream with crushed green herbs

– Sauces and Toppings

Sometimes it takes a small step to make a standard dish into a fabulous meal. Below are some of our favorite sauces and toppings that can elevate any fish, pasta or meat to "the next level". These are homemade from simple and healthy ingredients, and will surprise you with how easy they are to make.

Our version of teriyaki sauce
Adjust quantities according to the number of portions you are making. This should be sufficient for two filets of salmon.
– 1 tbs soya sauce
– 1 tbs rice syrup
– 1 tbs Aivar (North Macedonian, Bosnian or Montenegrin pepper ketchup) or tomato ketchup
Warm/mix together to a thick paste to coat the fish, meat or vegetarian alternative
If possible, leave it in the fridge for a couple of hours, or until you are ready to cook.
Grill or bake in the oven.

Fresh Herb Sauce – Keeping it green
Either with a pestle and mortar or in a bowel, mix:
– Sea salt
– Crushed black pepper
– Fresh green herbs; parsley, dill, oregano, thyme, lemon rind, olive oil,

Rub on fish, meat or vegetarian alternative - and bake
Try to put them on your vegetables before roasting them.

Spicy Rub
– Salt
– Pepper
– Sweet paprika
– Sumac

Use any combination to enhance your fish, meat or vegetarian alternatives to give a gentle uplift to your meal. For a slightly stronger"kick", you can add either fresh chilli or dried chilli to any of the mixes. It is probably best not to add it to the green mix as it will detract from the fresh and fragrant flavour.

Crusty nut topping
Blend or crush any nut. We like hazelnuts, pistachio, walnuts, or pecans.
You can mix with breadcrumbs if you want.
To make the topping stick to the fish when you are grilling it, brush the fillets with either milk, oil, rice syrup, or egg white.

Olive tapenade
This makes a wonderful coating to fish, a sauce for pasta and it is amazing on bread. You can make your own by blitzing olives with either capers, or pine nuts, lemon rind or even anchovy (do remember these small fish are salty, so you will not need to add salt to this dish if you use them).

Pesto – easier than you might think
In a food processor mix:
– Any fresh herb
– Any nuts such as pine nuts, pistachio, hazelnuts
– Salt and pepper to taste
– Olive oil or any other oil such as hemp or walnut
Once ready, grate some fresh parmesan cheese.

Pesto is not just a pasta sauce – it can be added to soups, spread on fish or meat as a topping before baking, and even simply on a slice of bread – you will be amazed how fresh and tasty this can be.

Miso sauce

Miso paste is usually shop-bought, and not just used in oriental recipes. It can be a very versatile addition to your meal. Mix the paste with either soy sauce or water to make it easier to apply to the fish, chicken, vegetables, or tofu.

Rub in before baking or grilling.

Tahini Sauce

Tahini paste is a Mediterranean staple ingredient made from sesame seeds. Sesame can be eaten raw, but it's usually made into tahini sauce – one of the most common side dishes or dressings in any middle eastern table.

You can use tahini as a sauce for fish, meat or vegetables.
– 1tbs Tahini paste
– 1tbs Soya sauce
– Fresh pepper
– Paprika or sumac
– Za'atar
– Fresh herbs such as **parsley**, or **oregano**

– Vegetables as a main course

You should try and have a **couple** of **vegetarian meals** every week.

Aubergine

Score the aubergine and use either the miso sauce or Tahini sauce as a marinade, leave for an hour before baking.

Cauliflower steak

Cutting the cauliflower from the middle will give you a nice rounded large surface to cover and bake.

Stuffed vegetables

Peppers

Large mushrooms

These make a wonderful vessel to stuff with rice, quinoa, other chopped or grated vegetables. You can lightly fry and mix together. You can seal with a piece of cheese which will melt on top.

See the **"Stuffed Red Peppers"** recipe for a good example.

Vegetable Bake

An alternative to quiche or pie, which are pastry based, you can improvise and use e.g. grated celeriac as a base. Grate your choice of vegetables and mix with egg to bind together. Top with other vegetables or mixed pulses.

You can create a cheesy topping by mixing cream cheese, grated cheese, and bake in the oven until golden.

Soups

Soups are amazing all year round, but our favorite time to eat them is certainly in the winter, when a bowl of soup can keep you both full and warm. In our family we name soups by their color, making mealtime fun and creative.

You can substitute a variety of vegetables depending on what you have at home or what you can buy according to the season, making sure it's fresh.

How to make soup

Chop up your vegetables lightly, fry in a small amount of oil, add a stock cube and cover with boiling water.

Cook until soft. At this point you can start to add seasoning to taste, adding fresh herbs such as parsley, sage, basil and/or dill.

You can blend all your vegetables together. To create a thick and creamy soup, add water to your preferred consistency.

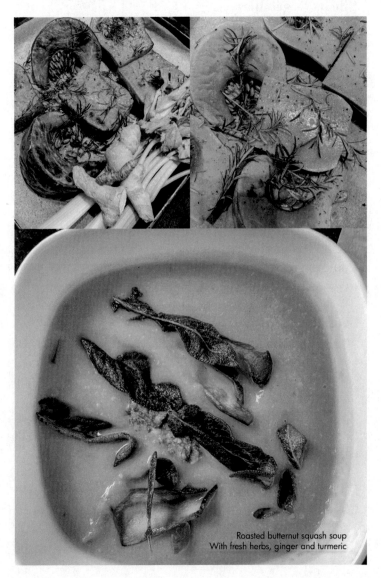

Roasted butternut squash soup
With fresh herbs, ginger and turmeric

Last Word

We are what we eat – is not just a proverb, rather an opportunity to reinvent ourselves. Cooking is not a chore, but rather a creative, expressive opportunity to have fun.

You don't have to be a chef when you cook – just follow some of the ideas presented, and in no time you'll find yourself immersed in a world of fresh flavors and experiences that will transform your meals, and help you to boost your immune system and stay healthy.

Fish wrapped in rice paper
Serves 2

Ingredients
2 fillets of fish
rice paper - soaked and ready to use

Dressing
1 tbs sesame oil
1 tbs light soy sauce
1 tsp yuzu juice
rind of 1 lime
1tsp grated ginger
1 tsp grated fennel
1 small chilli
fresh green herbs such as parsley, fennel leaves

Method
Mix all the dressing ingredients together.
Drizzle on top of the fish.
Wrap in rice paper.
Bake in the oven (200 °C) for 10 minutes.

Serve with
Mixed vegetable stir-fry or other green leaves, such as spinach or rainbow chard.

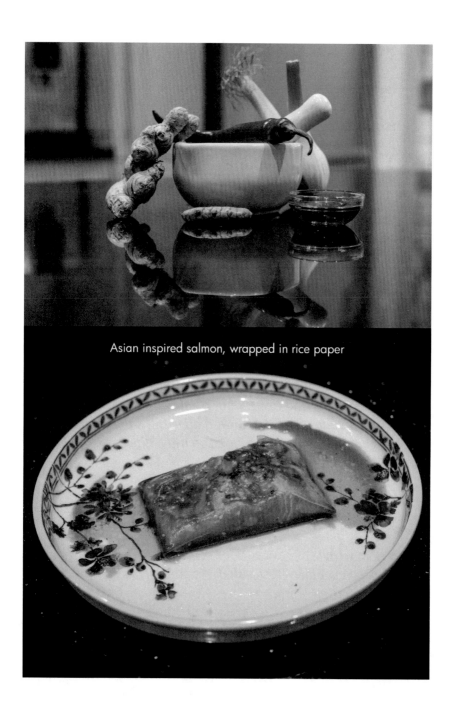

Asian inspired salmon, wrapped in rice paper

Whole mackerel roasted with fresh herbs

Serves 2

Ingredients
2 whole mackerel fish (or any other you prefer)

Stuffing
Any seasonal fresh herbs e.g:
Rosemary
Thyme
Oregano
Dill
Parsley
Fresh lemons
Olive Oil
Salt and pepper

Method
Mix all herbs and insert into the gut of the fish. Place the fish in a baking tray. Drizzle with olive oil, salt and pepper.
You can add more of the herbs on top of the fish as well as the sliced lemons.
Cover the tray with foil and bake in oven (200 °C) for 12 minutes. Remove the foil and cook for further few minutes to crisp.

Serve with
Mixed vegetable, fresh salad, rice or potatoes

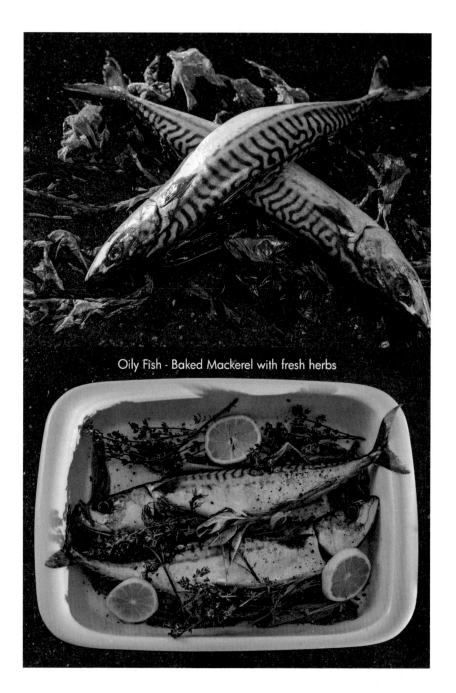

Oily Fish - Baked Mackerel with fresh herbs

Asian-inspired chicken strips

Serves 2

Ingredients
500g chicken or turkey breast
Cut the meat into small strips, or buy ready-made

Sauce
2tbs soya sauce
2tbs honey or rice syrup or maple syrup
2tbs red wine
¼ of a fresh chilli, thinly diced
¼ thumb of fresh ginger, diced small
¼ tsp pepper

Method
Put all the sauce ingredients in a small pan and gently heat till it bubbles.
Leave to cool.
Line a baking tray with baking paper and place the chicken or turkey on the tray and pour the sauce evenly on top.
Leave to marinate for a few hours or overnight in the fridge.
Once ready to cook, place in the oven at 190 to 200 °C for 15-20 minutes.
Ensure chicken is cooked well. It should come out white when cut in the middle.

Serve with
Rice or potatoes
Boiled green beans or bok choy
Purple-sprouting broccoli
Carrots

Mediterranean-style baked chicken

Serves 2

Ingredients
4 chicken thighs
1 small aubergine
1 sweet red pepper
1 red onion, (can replace with celery and carrots)
200g courgettes (zucchini)
For the marinade
10 sun-dried tomatoes
A handful of fresh basil leaves
A handful of fresh oregano
Zest of a lemon
1 clove of garlic (optional)
2tbs of olive oil

Method
Blend the marinade ingredients together, resembling a pesto consistency (if too thick, add more olive oil) and set aside.
Cut all the vegetables into chunks.
Use 1tbs of the marinade and mix into the vegetables.
Spread the rest of the marinade on the chicken.
Line a baking tray with baking paper and put the vegetables on top and layer with the chicken.
Sprinkle with salt and black pepper to taste.
Cover with aluminium foil and bake in the oven at 190 °C for approximately 35 minutes.
Check that the chicken is cooked well before serving.

Serve with
Rice or potatoes

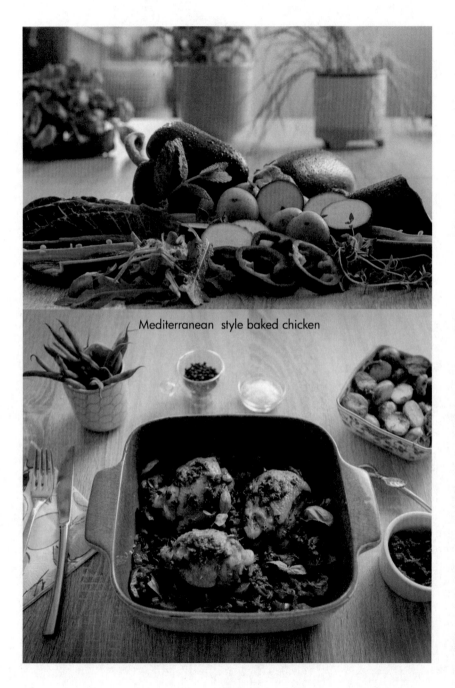

Mediterranean style baked chicken

Chicken with mushroom sauce

Serves 2

Ingredients
200g of chicken breast, cut into strips
2tbs of plain white flour
For the sauce:
200-300g of mixed mushrooms
¼ cup of white or red wine
1 small shallot
A handful of mixed fresh herbs: such as rosemary, sage, oregano, basil, parsley.

Method
In a big frying pan, cut the shallots and lightly fry with either olive oil or rapeseed oil, please remember that olive oil should be used at lower temperatures. Then cut and chop the mushrooms and season with salt and pepper.

Once the mushrooms have started to color, add the wine and leave to evaporate for a couple of minutes. Add all the chopped mixed herbs, mix it well and fry for another couple of minutes. Move to another dish and set aside.

Place the chicken or turkey strips in a sealed plastic bag with the flour and shake till the chicken is covered.

In the same frying pan, fry the coated chicken strips for 5-10 minutes.
Then pour the mushroom sauce on top of the chicken and heat till ready to serve.

Serve with
Green beans
Wilted spinach
Baked sweet potato
Feel free to add fresh rocket leaves.

Baked lamb chops in a herb crust

Serves 2

Ingredients
1-2 chops per person, depending on size
Remove all excess fat prior to cooking
Herb Crust
A handful of fresh basil
A handful of fresh parsley
A handful of pine nuts
¼ cup of olive oil

Method
Blend the herb crust ingredients together until resembling a pesto-like consistency, then add salt and pepper to taste.

Coat the lamb chops on both sides with the fresh herb sauce, with any herby leftovers set aside. Line a baking tray with baking paper and place the chops on top. Bake in the oven for approximately 8 minutes on each side at 190 °C.

Serve with
Fresh salad: lettuce and rocket with a lemon and olive oil dressing
Boiled new potatoes: cut the potatoes in half and add the rest of the herb sauce, once cooked
Roasted vegetables: such as red peppers and aubergines.

Beef skewers

Serves 2

Ingredients
200-300g of beef, cut into chunks or pre-brought
Variety of vegetables cut to similar sizes to place between the chunks of meat
For the marinade
2tbs soya sauce
2tbs Worcestershire sauce
2tbs balsamic vinegar
2tbs vegetable oil
Black pepper

Method
Mix all the sauce ingredients together
Arrange the meat and vegetables on a skewer in alternating order until full.
With a kitchen brush, coat the skewer with the sauce.
Line a baking tray with baking paper and place the skewers on top.
Bake at 190 °C for 15 minutes, rotating the skewers from time to time.

Serve with
A fresh salad of mixed leaves with diced avocado and dressing of lemon and olive oil
A warm tomato and bean salad (see separate recipe)

Warm tomato and bean salad

Serves 2

Ingredients
A can of mixed beans, such as borlotti beans
2 Roma tomatoes
A handful of cherry tomatoes
¼- ½ fresh chilli
A handful of fresh parsley
1 fresh fennel
Sesame seeds
Fresh thyme

Method
Cut the Roma tomato into quarters, and quarter the fennel.
Cut the cherry tomatoes into half and place in a baking tray with the fennel and Roma tomatoes.
Drizzle with olive oil, sesame seeds, fresh thyme, and fresh parsley and roast for 8-10 minutes at 190 °C.
Wash and rinse the beans.
Add the roasted fennel and tomatoes to the beans with all the juices from the oven.
Season with olive oil, salt, pepper, and fresh lemon juice.
Decorate with fresh parsley.

Serve with
Crusty bread or crackers

Celeriac pie

Serves 2

Ingredients
1 celeriac
200g spinach
1 can/400g of precooked lentils
200g of cream cheese (any alternatives will do)
100g grated cheddar (strong) cheese
50g parmesan
2 whole eggs
Salt
Pepper

Method
Grate the celeriac and chop the spinach, mix together.
Wash and rinse the lentils and combine them into the mixture.
In a separate bowl, beat the eggs, fold in the grated cheeses and cream cheese. Season with salt and pepper.
Add the vegetable mixture to the egg mixture and fold together gently.

In an oiled, ovenproof dish pour the combined mixture and sprinkle with extra cheese and grated nutmeg or flaked almonds (if desired) and bake 200 °C for 20 minutes or until golden brown.

Serve with
Fresh green salad: with dill and cucumber
Roasted red peppers or roasted tomatoes

Stuffed red peppers

Serves 2

Ingredients
2 large red peppers
50g uncooked quinoa
2 courgettes (zucchini)
2 carrots
1 tomato sliced
75-80g sliced goats' cheese

Method
Cut the peppers into halves and deseed, sprinkle with olive oil, and roast for 5-10 minutes to soften the peppers.

In the meantime, cook the quinoa and in a frying pan, fry the grated courgettes and carrots with olive oil until soft.

Mix the cooked quinoa and the vegetables.

Stuff the peppers with the mixture.

Season to taste.

You can add fresh herbs such as basil, thyme, or sage.

Top with slices of fresh tomato and goat cheese.

Bake in the oven at 190 °C for 10 minutes or until cheese is melted on top.

before serving.

Serve with
Bed of cooked spinach
Green beans
Mash potato or any mashed vegetable

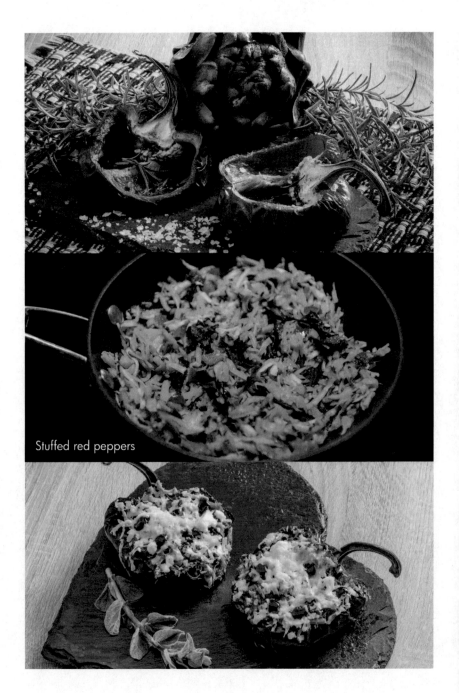

Stuffed red peppers

Miso aubergine

Serves 2

Ingredients
2 aubergines
2tbs miso paste
2tbs soya sauce
Fresh ground pepper
Sprinkle of sesame seeds or flaked almonds

Method
Cut the aubergines in half (lengthwise) and with a knife create a criss-cross on the top layer of the aubergine in a diagonal pattern.

In a bowl combine the miso, soya and fresh ground pepper. If the paste seems too thick add a dash of water, mix together.

With a kitchen brush coat the aubergine with the sauce, ensuring you go into the diagonal criss-cross.

Sprinkle with sesame seeds or flaked almonds and add a few drops of sesame oil.

Leave to rest for an hour before baking in the oven at 190 °C for about 20 minutes or until brown on top.

Serve with
Bok choy
Broccoli
Fresh salad
Rice with fried beansprouts

Note: This can also be applied to cauliflower that you cut lengthwise, to create the appearance of a cauliflower steak, or sweet potato and parsnips.

Tofu

Serves 2

Ingredients
A packet of extra-firm tofu: roughly 250g
1tsp grated ginger or a small thumb of fresh ginger
1tbs soya sauce
1 small fresh chilli
½ tps of five-spice
Sprinkle of sesame seeds
1tbs olive oil
½ tbs sesame seed oil

Method
Cut and cube the tofu and pat off the excess water.

In a frying pan add olive oil and fresh chilli, ginger, and five-spice: flavouring the oil. Then add the tofu once the oil is hot.

Once the tofu absorbs the oil, sprinkle again with sesame seed oil.

When the tofu is beginning to crisp, lower the temperature and add the soya sauce.

Sprinkle with sesame seeds.

Serve with
Mixed vegetable stir fry
Rice or rice noodles

Crispy Tofu

Serves 2

Ingredients
200g firm tofu - pressed and drained
1 tbs vegetable oil
spice rub
1tbs cornflour
1/2 tbs flour
1 tbs ground ginger
1 tbs paprika
salt and pepper

Method
Cut tofu into cubes (you can choose how big).
Mix all dry ingredients together to a dry rub.
Cover the tofu pieces in the dry rub (coating the tofu).
Fry in vegetable oil, until all sides are crispy.

Serve with
carrot "noodles" – see recipe below

Carrot Noodles

Serves 2

Ingredients
4 Carrots
Fresh ginger
Stick of celery
1 tbs soy sauce
1tbs olive oil

Method
Peel the carrots into long strips with a potato peeler. Heat the oil. Add the celery and ginger, Add the carrots and cook till soft. Add soy sauce halfway through.

Serve with
Steamed spinach or green beans

Grilled Courgette (Zucchini) Flowers

Serves 2

Ingredients
Two courgette flowers
One courgette – finely grated,
A few basil leaves
Tbs olive oil
2 tbs cream, or crème fresh, if desired. (can be excluded)
Salt and pepper to taste.

Method
In a pan on a low heat, fry the grated courgette in olive oil, season to taste.
Add the basil leaves: you can tear them by hand into small pieces.
Optional: once cooked, add the cream and remove from the heat and allow to cool down.

Stuff the flowers with the fried courgette, twist the flower at the top, to create a seal.
Drizzle with olive oil, bake on a low heat 180c for 5 min.
Serve warm.

Serve with
Mozzarella Salad – see below

Mozzarella Salad (Caprese Plus)

Serves 2

Ingredients
Mozzarella cheese
Thinly sliced beef tomato
Slices of avocado
Basil leaves
Olive oil
Option – balsamic vinegar

Method
Slice tomato and avocado to your choice of thickness. Arrange on a plate and top with mozzarella cheese. You can tear the mozzarella, as well as the basil. If preferred, you can cut both ingredients instead. Sprinkle with olive oil and optionally with balsamic vinegar. This salad will also accompany white fish, such as sea bream or sea bass.

Serve with
Bread, crackers, or pasta

Mixed Vegetable Pasta

Serves 2

Ingredients
150g dry linguine
10-12 cherry tomatoes, halved
roasted sweet potatoes or butternut squash, cubed
1/2 avocado (optional)
handful basil leaves
handful thin green beans, cooked in water
2 tbsp single cream

Method
Cook your pasta as instructed on the pack.

While the pasta is cooking: in a pan, add olive oil and lightly fry the sweet potato, tomatoes and thin green beans.

Add 2tbs cream, basil, and 1tbs of pasta water, then add the drained pasta and mix.

Thinly cut the avocado and add to the pasta dish – mix.

Grate some fresh Parmesan on top and serve.

Serve with
Side salad

Green eggs (no ham) – Green Shakshuka

Serves 2-4

Ingredients
200g Swiss rainbow chard (separate stalks from leaves but use both)
100g kale
200g fresh spinach
2 celery sticks
4 eggs
100ml of cream (any alternatives)
Salt
Pepper
1tbs olive oil
Variety of green herbs: such as parsley, coriander, oregano, thyme, lemon balm, or sage.

Method
In a large frying pan heat the oil and add chopped celery and the chopped Swiss chard (just the stalks). Fry until soft.

Add all the leaves, torn to small pieces, either by hand or chopped by a knife.
Add to the frying pan and mix well. Season with salt and pepper.
Add the cream and fresh green herbs.

Once soft, create four wells in the pan and break the eggs into the wells.
Cook to the preferred consistency of the egg.
Grate parmesan on top and sprinkle with fresh herbs.

Serve with
Fresh bread
Chopped vegetable salad of tomato, cucumber, and lettuce

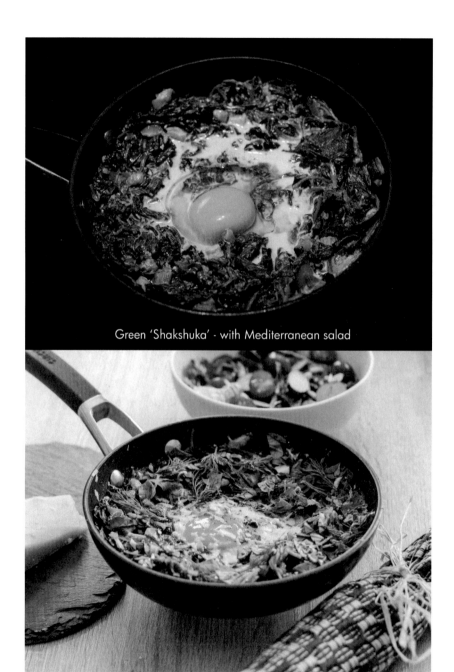

Green 'Shakshuka' - with Mediterranean salad

Farinata (Chickpea Pancake)

Serves 2

Ingredients
1 cup chickpea flour
2 cups water
2tbs olive oil
1tsp salt
Optional – rosemary or za'atar

Method
Add all the ingredients to a bowl and whisk until frothy
Rest for 1 hour
Grease a large thin dish and pour the wet batter in, optionally sprinkle with fresh rosemary or za'atar.

Bake 190°C for 40 minutes (until the top begins to brown), then let it cool.
For a light meal serve with fresh salad or alternatively use instead of carbohydrates for your main course, such as potatoes.

Serve with
Fresh salad or as an alternative to bread

Homemade Granola

Ingredients
4 cups of oats
1 1/2 cup of mixed nut (chopped almonds, pecans, hazel-nuts and walnuts)
1 cup of mixed seeds (pumpkin, flax seeds, hemp seeds)
1tsp of salt
1 tbs cinnamon
1/2 cup of oil (hemp seed oil, walnut oil)
1/2 cup of maple syrup + little bit of rice syrup if you want big clusters
1 tsp vanilla extract
dried fruit/ additional toppings.

Method
Mix the oats, nuts, seeds, salt and cinnamon in a bowl. Stir well to combine. Add more nuts or seeds if desired.
Pour the oil, maple syrup, rice syrup and vanilla on to the mix and stir to combine thoroughly.
Line a baking tray with baking paper and spread evenly.
Bake at 170 °C (fan) for 20-25 minutes.
Stir halfway- pile on to each other for larger clusters.
Take out of the oven and leave to rest.
Once cooled, mix in the additional toppings.

Serve with
Yoghurt, milk of your choice or as a topping for ice cream or crumble

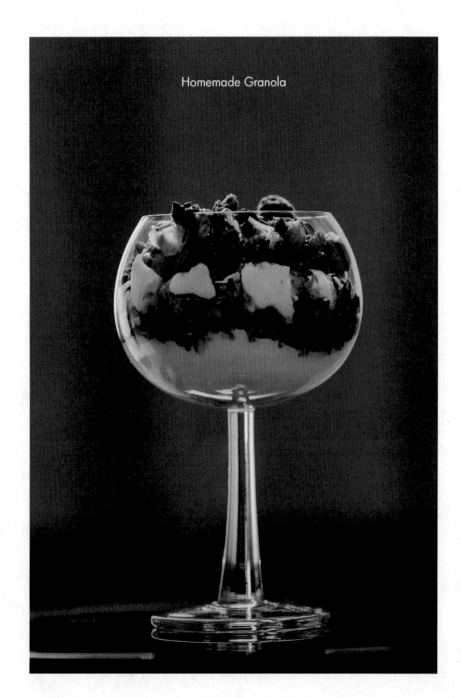

Homemade Granola

Desserts and Puddings

Not always the naughty one... these can be made with some healthy options such as fruit, which are good for providing antioxidants, and cocoa powder, which is also high in iron.

Blueberry Crumb Cake

Ingredients
Base
125g plain flour (any flour will do)
1 1/2 tsp of baking powder
50g butter
1/4 tsp salt
80g sugar
1 egg
75ml of milk (any alternative will do)
juice of half a lemon
300g blueberry (frozen)
Topping
75g oats/flour
80g sugar
57g butter
1/2 tsp of cinnamon
zest of 1/2 or 1 lemon.
any seeds you wish to add

Method
Whisk the dry base ingredients together.
In a separate bowl, beat butter and sugar together then add the egg and lemon juice till smooth.
Pour the dry mixture and the milk into the smooth mixture in small batches, and beat till smooth.
To make the crumble topping, add all of the ingredients in a bowl and crumble/rub together to reach your desired consistency.
Grease a small tin, pour the base mixture in, then add the frozen blueberries, and finally - top with the crumble topping.
Bake at 180°C for 35 minutes.

Flip the cake and again bake upside down for 5-10 mins, until the bottom of it is nice and crispy.
Flip again and serve.

Berry Crumble

Ingredients
500g of frozen mixed berries
50g of sugar or rice syrup or maple syrup
50g butter
90g flour of your choice
1/2 tsp of ground cinnamon
any mixed seeds you want

Method
Grease a baking tray.
Spread the berries at the bottom of the tray.
Add the rest of the ingredients in a bowl and rub together to form your crumble topping.
Spread over the berries.
Bake at 180 °C for 20-25 minutes until the crumble is golden on top.

Serve with
Greek style yoghurt

Rhubarb Dish

Ingredients
4/5 stalks of rhubarb
2/3 tbs of sugar or maple syrup
base
1 cup of oats
1/2 cup of mixed seeds
1 tsp coco powder
1tsp cinnamon

Method
Grease a baking tray.
Spread all the base ingredients together mixing slightly at the bottom.
Drizzle with maple syrup (around half the overall quantity).
Cut up the stalks of rhubarb (roughly 5cm) and place on top to cover everything.
Drizzle with water and sprinkle with the remaining sugar or maple syrup.
Bake at 180 °C for 20 minutes or until rhubarb is soft (stab with a fork to test).

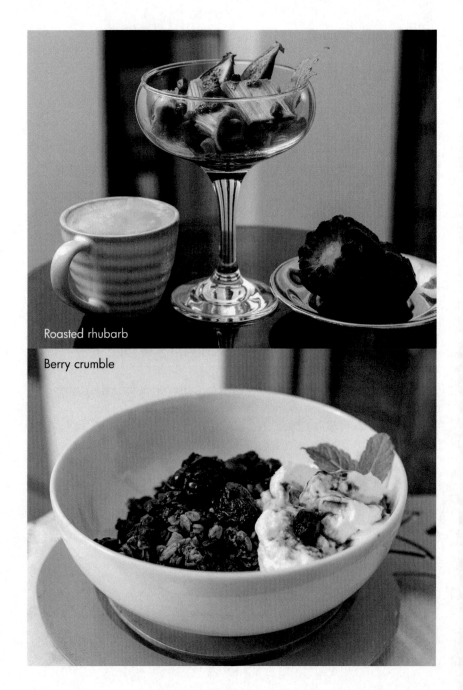

Roasted rhubarb

Berry crumble

88

Tahini Biscuits

Ingredients
1 cup tahini
1 cup sugar
3 cups flour or flour alternatives
1/2 cup sesame oil
1 tsp vanilla extract
optional: cinnamon, coco powder,

Method
Mix all the ingredients together until smooth.
Line a baking tray with baking paper.

Scoop 1tbsp of mixture on the tray for each biscuit – leave space between.
Bake 190°C for 10 minutes until golden brown.

Multicolored Gooseberry Tray Bake

Ingredients
400-500g of mixed gooseberries
40g sugar
tsp cinnamon
tsp vanilla extract
200g almond flour
80g caster sugar
3 egg whites
50g of unsalted butter
1/2 cup walnut oil

Method
Cut the gooseberries in half, and sprinkle with cinnamon and the 40g of sugar and vanilla extract.
Cover and shake it well, set aside.
Whisk the egg whites till fluffy, but not meringue like, then whisk in all the dry ingredients.
Add the oil and melted butter, lightly whisk.
Oil a baking tray.
Pour the batter in, and add the gooseberry mixture on top.
Bake at 185°C for 40 minutes, then cover with silver foil and bake for another 10 minutes.

Serve with
Greek style yoghurt

Small Black Sesame Seed Cake

Ingredients
36g black sesame seeds
20g sesame seed oil
50g brown sugar
1 egg
100ml coconut milk
90g oat crème fraiche
100g rice flour
1tsp baking powder

Method
Pulse the sesame seeds to create a paste, (you can dry fry them before for a richer, deeper flavour).

Add the paste to a bowl and whisk in the sugar, oil, egg, milk and crème fraiche. Then add the dry ingredients and mix in.

Pour into a greased pan and sprinkle with mixed sesame seeds.

Bake at 170 °C for 1 hour and then rest for 1 hour before serving.

Matcha Mochi

Ingredients
185g rice flour
2 tsp sugar
1/2 tsp baking powder
2 tsp matcha powder (you can add more if you like the taste or you feel you need)
1 cup water
3/4 cup coconut milk
1tsp vanilla extract

Method
Whisk flour, sugar, baking powder and match in a bowl.
Separately blend water, milk and vanilla extract.
Pour the wet ingredients into the dry ingredients and whisk until smooth.
Grease a baking pan and pour the mocha mixture into it.
Cover tightly with aluminium foil.
Bake at 130°C for 60-80 minutes.
Remove the foil and allow to cool.
Cut into equal-sized cubes.

GLOSSARY

Aivar: a Balkan pepper ketchup, made from sweet, roasted peppers – popular throughout all the Balkan countries. Recipes vary from country to country, but we use North Macedonian, Bosnian or Montinegrin varieties in our recipes.

Avocado: botanically a large pear-shaped fruit, containing a single large seed. The avocado has green flesh, contains monounsaturated fatty acids and a variety of vitamins. The flesh can be eaten raw or used in a variety of recipes.

Basil: a culinary herb, used in Mediterranean cooking. It has a sweet flavour and aroma. Contains a variety of vitamins and minerals. A part of the mint family.

Celeriac: a type of root vegetable, generally a brown, round bulb. It has a distinctive taste that has a nutty, celery-like flavour.

Fennel: the leaves are a highly aromatic herb (similar to liquorice). The white bulb can be used in a variety of recipes. The nutrients in the fennel are linked to a range of health benefits.

FODMAP stands for "**F**ermentable **O**ligo-, **D**i-, **M**ono-saccharides **A**nd **P**olyols". These are a type of carbohydrate or sugar that do not get absorbed easily by the gut in some people. They may find their way to the lower reaches of the gut, where they can act as a fuel for gut bacteria - and produce uncomfortable gas as a result. Their presence in the intestine may cause diarrhoea, particularly in those people who have irritable bowel syndrome.

Common FODMAPs include:
– Fructose: a simple sugar found in many fruits and vegetables.
– Lactose: a sugar which is found in dairy products like milk.
– Fructans: found in many foods, including grains like wheat, spelt, rye and barley.
– Galactans: found in large amounts in legumes, like peas and beans (the cause of wind in many people).
– Polyols: these are sugar-like alcohols, which include xylitol, sorbitol, maltitol and mannitol. They are found in certain fruits and vegetables and some of them are used as artificial sweeteners, including in chewing gum and certain candies.

Maple Syrup: a syrup obtained from the sap of maple trees, sweet in flavour; it can replace honey or sugar in many recipes. Acceptable sweetener in a low FODMAP diet.

Microbiome: there are over 100 trillion bugs in or on our bodies. Most of these microrganisms live in our gut, and for the most part, in the large intestine. We have learned to live in harmony with them from the moment we are born.

These microbes are collectively called the microbiome and consist of bacteria, fungi, protozoa and viruses – we have as much as 2kg of bugs which help digest our food, have a role in strengthening our immune systems and also producing vitamins, such as B12, thiamine, riboflavin and Vitamin K, (which is needed for healthy blood clotting when we cut ourselves, for example).

Miso: traditional Japanese seasoning produced by fermenting soya beans, rice, barley or seaweed. The result is a thick paste used for sauces and spreads or to make a soup.

Oregano: a herb used in many Mediterranean dishes. It is from the mint family, containing antioxidants; it has antiviral and antibacterial properties.

Pesto: a sauce, traditionally consisting of crushed basil leaves, garlic, and pine nuts, blended with olive oil. However, you can add or substitute any leaves, herbs, nuts, or other spices.

Rice syrup: a sweetener that can be used to substitute sugar or honey. It can be used in a low FODMAP diet. The main component is glucose.

Sumac: a ground spice made from the red berries of a wild bush grown in Mediterranean climates. It is used as a spice in many Middle Eastern dishes. The powder has a lemony flavour.

Tahini: A Mediterranean sesame paste

Za'atar: a blend of savoury dried herbs such as oregano and thyme, mixed with sesame seeds. Used in many Middle Eastern dishes. It has a warm, earthy, salty flavour.

PART 3

Exercise and Fitness

A HEALTHY BODY

The key to a healthy body is understanding the harmony between a good diet and a body that is in good physical shape. A good physical shape includes different factors: balance, flexibility, muscular strength – essential to maintain a correct posture – and a healthy heart. Many people think that exercise is difficult or uninteresting, or perhaps a luxury, but with a little thought, a routine can be incorporated even into the busiest of lives. The key is that exercise doesn't have to be complex, but it does have to be achievable – and the importance of training in equal measure flexibility, balance, and good posture, which is essential for the elderly, should be ingrained in younger people who may take their physical health for granted.

Working in line with a healthy immune system and balanced diet, exercise is imperative in maintaining a strong body. People with all levels of fitness should be able to do some of the exercises and postures that we suggest in this chapter. We have made them adjustable to any situation, as they can all be done in small spaces at home or outdoors – so there is no need to go to a gym. Some of the exercises can be practiced gradually increasing the level of challenge as the body adapts and becomes stronger and more flexible. Listen to your body and attempt at least to develop the first posture and exercises shown.

It is important to emphasise that the brain perceives exercise positively because physical activity produces hormones called **"endorphins"**, which help our mental health and make us feel happy. These hormones help the immune system, while exercise itself reduces stress, by helping reduce unnecessary surges of stress-related hormones, such as adrenaline (which can have an adverse effect on our immune system and our health).

Everything needs to be balanced, as too much exercise is also not good, because the body needs time to recover. Exercise can be done anywhere, but remember that, as with everything else, it should be done in moderation.

1) Posture

Correct postural alignment is imperative for a healthy body. Putting it simply, bad posture will wear your body out, leaving muscles and joints strained and fatigued. However, correcting your posture will help to keep your nerves, blood vessels, muscles, ligaments, and tendons healthy. In most cases, it is never too late to correct your posture – even a severely bad posture can be greatly improved in 30 days. For most of us, staring at screens, typing away at a desk (or even typing on the sofa) has become part of our daily life and work. The temptation to naturally slump over must be resisted! If working on a computer, it is best to work sitting on a chair, with your shoulder blades against the back of the chair.

STANDING POSTURE TIPS
– Push down through heels trying to get taller
– Bring hips slightly back, directly above heels
– Top of head to the ceiling, relax chin, elongating
– Open chest, shoulders back

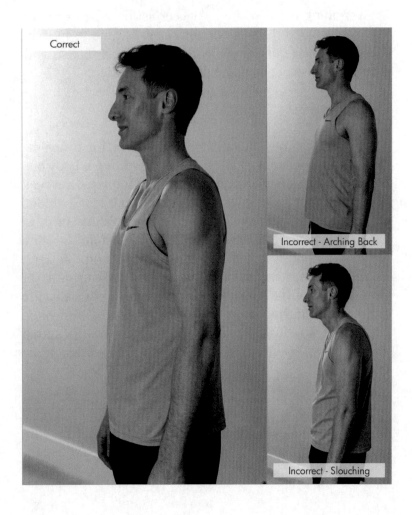

Correct

Incorrect - Arching Back

Incorrect - Slouching

2) The Warm-Up Routine ("Cardio")

Warming up the body helps it to prepare for exercise by accelerating the flow of blood as it courses through the cardiovascular system (heart and blood vessels). This raises the body's temperature and increases blood flow to the muscles. Warming up is also our best bet to avoid injury.

*Start with 30 seconds on each exercise, then 1 min, building to 1min 30sec on each for more advanced fitness levels:

– **Jogging on the spot**
– **Jumping jacks**

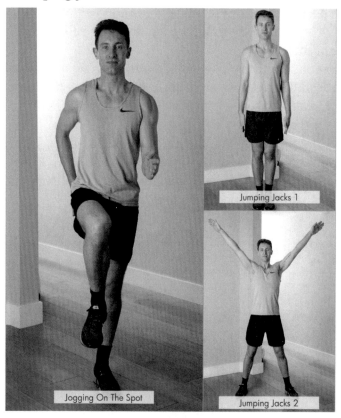

Jumping Jacks 1

Jumping Jacks 2

Jogging On The Spot

– Burpees

This has an odd name and sounds rather complicated, but burpees are actually quite simple once you get the hang of them:

1) Start with the body in a squatting position with knees bent, back straight, and feet comfortably shoulder-width apart.

2) Lower hands to the floor in front of you so they are just inside your feet (see illustration).

3) With the bodyweight sent to your hands, kick your feet backwards, so you are now both on your hands and toes, and in a pushup position (see illustration).

4) Keep the body straight from head to heels and then do one pushup.

5) Follow this by a "frog" kick by jumping your feet forwards to where they started at the beginning of the exercise.

6) Stand and reach your arms over your head, as if stretching for the sky.

7) Jump quickly into the air so you land back where you started (see illustration).

8) As soon as you land with knees bent, get back into a squat position and do another repetition.

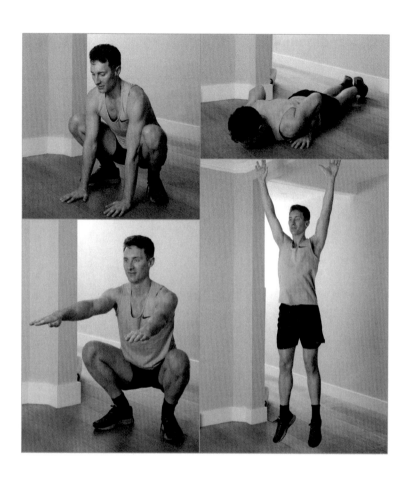

3) Conditioning

Conditioning exercises build a stronger and more flexible body. It is not only "cardio" that helps the body to lose weight - conditioning is essential for weight loss (stronger muscles will burn more calories) and help in building a balanced and stable physique.

– **Lunges/squats**, 10 lunges on each side, 10 squats

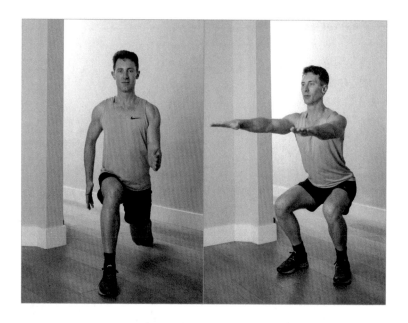

– Press-ups, 10 repetitions in each position

3 variations:

a) Wide
b) Narrow
c) Diamond

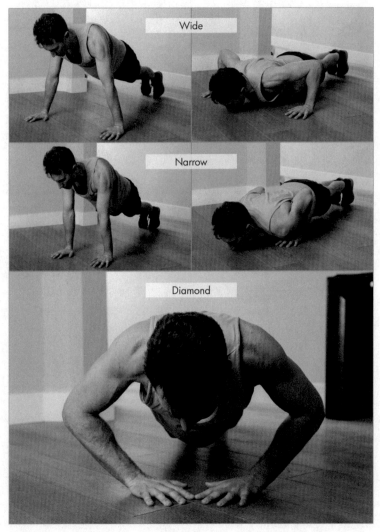

– **Mountain climbers**, 20 repetitions

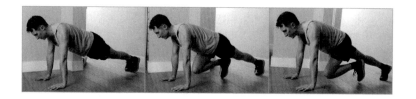

– Arms and Shoulders, 10 repetitions on each arm
a) Arm curls
b) Side lateral raises

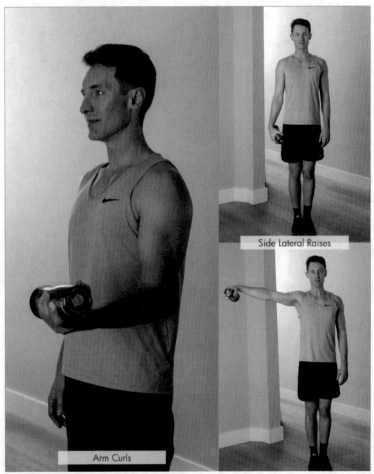

Side Lateral Raises

Arm Curls

4) Balance

Balance is what is needed to control and maintain a desired position in the environment. Balance is controlled by the brain and specifically requires the engagement of the core muscles in the body, such as the abdominals. Even to stand up straight, we need a significant degree of balance, even if we do not realize it (remember that toddler trying to walk for the first time!). More advanced postures and balances need more core engagement. For example, try standing on one leg and raising up the standing heel (so that you are balancing on the toes of one foot). This is a good example of when we activate core engagement to keep us from falling. The taller we stand on one leg and the more balanced we are, the more the core will be engaged.

Improving balance comes from focusing. Take your time on the postures outlined below, increasing the duration of the stance as you gain strength.

– Plank position

*Start with 30 seconds on each, then 1 min, building to 1 min and 30 sec on each for more advanced fitness levels.

a) Two hands
b) Two hands, one leg off the floor
c) Side plank, one hand off the floor

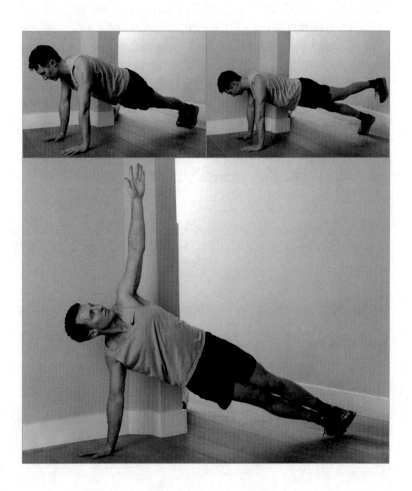

5) Stretching

Stretching is a must after all exercise routines, including extended walking. Even without exercise, we should aim to stretch three times a week. Stretching improves posture, the range of motion and it also decreases muscle soreness, especially back pain. The exercises outlined below will increase blood flow to the muscles, shorten recovery time and help with general relaxation and easing of the mind.

*Hold each position for 20 seconds, deepening the stretch and intensity when you can.

– **Touching toes** (this is a fantastic stretch for all levels. Anyone will be able to get more flexibility and have their hands closer to the floor if his exercise is done every day.)

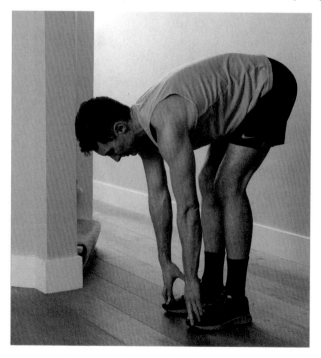

– Lunge
a) Front lunge
b) Front lunge, hand on the floor
c) Front lunge, hand on the floor, other raised up

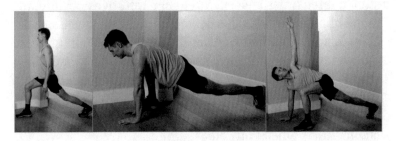

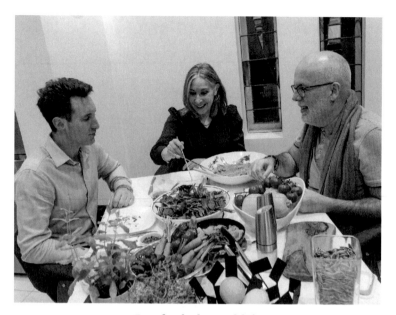

Lead a balanced life

Index